How to Keep Your Metabolism Burning Like a Furnace

I0422182

This is a workout & diet plan designed for the average American, who is busy, and perhaps lazy, and wants the most efficient and effective means of achieving the desired muscle mass and fat-burning potential that will give the physique and level of health desired in life.

A disciplined exercise and diet routine can be a major component in achieving health, not only on a physical level, but also on a psychological and emotional level.

This booklet is dedicated to the average American, to whom it is directed, in gratitude to our Founding Fathers, to the soldiers who fought for our freedom and to God who has given us all we have.

May we be able to use our hard won freedom to benefit ourselves, our communities and our nation in ways that glorifies God.

ORDERING NEW COPIES
Copies can be ordered at:
1. CREATESPACE.COM - https://www.createspace.com/5462660
2. AMAZON.COM
Use the discount code at Createspace.com to save $3 (WX93GCLY)

TABLE OF CONTENTS

About the Author

Matthew Wilk lives a celibate life in the Ann Arbor, Michigan area. He has a B.S. in Civil Engineering from Michigan State University in East Lansing, Michigan and an almost completed B.A. in Philosophy from Sacred Heart Major Seminary in Detroit, Michigan. He has been perfecting an exercise and diet routine for 15 years as he attempts to live a disciplined life in anticipation of joining a religious order.

This book is a ready-made routine of exercises and diet principles intended for the average person who wants to develop a regular routine but does not want to do the research and experimentation necessary to determine what works best for them. It is intended to be for anyone within the normal range of age and weight, but can be used by those at the extremes as well, if they are willing. There is a workout routine for each day, upper body twice per week, lower body once per week and aerobic exercise three times per week. The diet principles consist of the five types of food groups to include in each meal, what a typical portion size should be and how much water to drink everyday. The diagrams in the second half of the book display the motions for each exercise and describe how to perform it most effectively. This workout and diet plan is meant simply as an aid to have more discipline in exercise and eating in order to maintain a desirable amount of physical strength, good internal health, and an attractive physique. It is aimed at obtaining the best results in a moderate amount of workout time and with simplicity in diet. It may be said that 90% of what most people want can be obtained with this plan, while avoiding an elaborate workout routine or a complicated nutrition plan.

The two things we desire most for our bodies are physical health and physical attractiveness. For a normal healthy body, the main requirements for maintenance are sleep, physical activity and nutrition. The latter two are the only ones that require an intentional effort to fulfill. Fortunately, if they are done well they can also be a means of achieving the other major desire for our bodies, physical attractiveness.

The object of this book is to provide a means of achieving that physical health and physical attractiveness in a way that is *effective*, getting us the result that we desire, and is *efficient*, reaching that result without going beyond the optimum expenditure of time and effort. As in anything else we do, we want the best return for our investment, and this is the goal of the plan in this book.

This plan is not a comprehensive explanation of theory on exercise or nutrition. Rather, it is the fruit of 15 years of experimentation and modification that provides a practical, ready-made routine that is enjoyable and stimulating and can be a staple in ones' life. This plan is intended for those who, either because of lack of interest or lack of time, do not want to wade through the vast array of exercise and diet resources but who simply want something that works and want something that can be started __today__ without the need of long hours of discernment and study.

For those of us who do not have the time or interest to get involved in elaborate workout routines or complicated diet requirements, but who still want good results, it is worth noting that probably 90% of what we want to achieve can be obtained by employing only a few principles and keeping a few simple routines. If you could get 90% of the same result as a complicated exercise and nutrition plan in considerably less time and effort (maybe 50% less) wouldn't it be worth it?

What you will find in this plan is a simple and effective way to:
1. Build muscle mass
2. Keep your metabolism burning calories
3. Stay healthy, flexible and strong

The principles and specific points of the plan are aimed at getting the best combination of results with a modest investment in order to get a high return for the energy spent. The emphasis is on simplicity so you can easily apply the principles and even take them with you wherever you go without needing a manual.

> ## THIS IS A **6-DAY-PER-WEEK** WORKOUT PLAN AND A **3-MEALS-A-DAY** DIET PLAN

What does it require?
  *Only a single set of dumbbells

The exercise routine is outlined for each day of the week. The simple diet plan is basically a *model* for you to apply wherever/whenever you cook or eat a meal. Both of these together are all you need in order to gain the physique and health you seek.

This system is meant for home, but is also simple enough to be portable - you can memorize the principles and exercises on your fingers and carry your dumbbells with you when you travel.

Along with seeking physical goals for our body, being disciplined with diet and exercise also has numerous psychological benefits. We don't normally identify them all but they range from higher energy level and higher self-esteem to better emotional balance and greater self-possession.

This plan is designed with simplicity, variety, efficiency, effectiveness and reasonableness in mind.

Workout Plan

The ideal exercise routine would be the one that gets you nearest the goal of the muscle development you seek and does so without sustaining any injuries. It is also desirable to complete the routine in an acceptable amount of time, and very important, is to enjoy oneself. The exercises chosen in this booklet are aimed at:

1. Working **all** of the major muscle groups in a **balanced** way
2. Working as **many** muscles as possible in as **few** exercises as possible
3. **Not overworking** any muscle group by working it more than once in a pronounced way.
4. Needing only **one set of dumbbells** and no machines or special equipment
5. Using **normal movements** of the joints and muscles involved for ease of form and to avoid unhealthy strain on muscles and joints

The major means of attaining muscle mass, a higher metabolic rate, and better physical health is through physical activity. Each type of activity serves a different purpose in maintaining health. The four focuses here are:

STRETCHING - For flexibility and blood flow
Weight Training:
UPPER BODY - For strength and mass building
LOWER BODY - For strength and toning
AEROBIC - For calorie-burning and increased heart rate

All of these together make up the 6-days-per-week exercise routine. The stretching is everyday and the other three are spread throughout the week.

In order to meet the desire for efficiency and convenience, the workout for each day is designed to be completed within 30-45 minutes.

Diet Plan

We can agree that the best diet is the one that provides the needed nutrition while avoiding foods that are unhealthy for you. Accomplishing this within the proper proportions and eating foods that you like are also key to being able to stick to the plan. The model diet arranged here is based on the following:

1. Providing all of the **major food groups and types of calories** in order to have the energy and nutrition for all the systems of the body
2. Allowing for **variety** within the food groups/types
3. Achieving **balanced** nutrition within reasonable proportions
4. Relying on **common** foods that are easily available at any grocery store
5. Having **regularity** of meal times and order in how and when meals are eaten

Proper nutrition and calorie intake can only happen by consuming the right foods in the right amounts. The five categories for eating healthy are:

MEAL INTAKE - Regularity and proportion for nutrition

WATER INTAKE - For blood flow and metabolic rate

FOODS TO AVOID - Minimize or eliminate unhealthy chemicals and substances from your body to feel healthier

SAUCES - To have things that add flavor and enjoyment

SUPPLEMENTS - How to get much more results in a quicker, easier way by taking a concentrated supplement

With the above areas of attention, keeping a regular 3-meals-a-day diet is easy and effective. Three meals a day is the basic idea, but snacks in between and feasting, especially on weekends or special occasions, can nicely round out overall eating practices.

Even among professionals in any field it is certain for a difference of opinions to exist, so it is also necessarily the case here that anything proposed is based on one interpretation of experience and what works. However, it is possible to avoid being overly scientific when developing something practical like an exercise routine because often times the limits of what you are working with can be known without a significant amount of study, such as what causes joint pain, what motions seem unnatural and how can a similar amount of work be accomplished in different ways.

The following design was arrived at by taking into account what many experts had to say as well as the results of trial and error during experimentation.

WEIGHT OF DUMBBELLS

- After some trial and error it was found that, for a beginner, using a weight that is about **10% of bodyweight for a typical male**, and about **5% of body weight for a typical female** is an effective amount of weight to build muscle mass and is a safe enough amount to avoid injury

> For example, a male of about *200 lbs.* could safely begin a workout routine using a weight of about *20 lbs.*

- Of course the amount of weight can be increased over time as greater strength develops, but the above starting weight is a *rule of thumb* that can be used in finding the first set of weights

NUMBER OF SETS & REPETITIONS

- Some experts recommend up to 5 or 6 sets per exercise, which is the ideal amount to reach the maximum growth potential, but since *it is the first few sets of the exercise that cause the bulk of the growth*, it is not necessary to have the additional sets unless you are really concerned about getting maximum muscle growth

- In other words, *the positive effect of adding additional sets diminishes* after the first few sets and becomes less and less the more that additional sets are added

For example, if the first three sets will get you about 90% of the same muscle growth as 6 sets, *we can stop at 3 sets and still get almost the same result*, thus saving time

• Experts recommend numbers of repetitions ranging from 6-10 reps for force, 10-15 reps for strength, and 15-20 reps for speed, but because of how light a weight is needed for beginners, it is easier to *make up for the lack of weight by having more reps*

• Likewise, *having more reps makes up for a lack of the number of sets*, so even though we only have three sets, we can still get a total of reps near what we would have had with more sets, e.g. 3 sets of 20 reps gives us the same as 5 sets of 12 reps

Therefore this plan recommends doing **3 sets at 20 reps per set** until strength increases or a change is desired with the plan, at which time a fewer number of reps can be substituted with a heavier weight

 ## MIXTURE OF WEIGHT-TRAINING AND AEROBIC EXERCISE

• Some experts recommend a two-week cycle with one week having upper body exercises twice and lower body once, and the second week having lower body twice and upper body once, both weeks having three days of aerobic activity along with it

In that schedule, there are three upper body days and three lower body days over a two week period, with six aerobic days, *that is not what we are doing here*

• The main reason for the above is that for a serious mass-building weight-training routine the muscles are supposed to have 4-5 days to recover between workouts, *but we do not need to go with the ideal*

• The upper body is worked a lot less in the modern post-farming economy and the lower body is already naturally large, only needs toning, and already gets worked in aerobics, so turning the routine into a one-week cycle affords greater simplicity and shifts the emphasis to a better balance:

Monday - Upper Body
Tuesday - Aerobic
Wednesday - Lower Body
Thursday - Aerobic
Friday - Upper Body
Saturday - Aerobic
Sunday - Rest

• In the above scheme, the muscles worked in the upper body still get *3-4 days of rest* between upper body workouts, and *one week* for lower

• The body needs a good amount of aerobic activity, about as much as muscle-building activity, so an *equal amount* of each is in the one-week cycle ...*3 days each of aerobic & muscle-building per week*

• Likewise, *one day of rest is needed every week* to recover physically and psychologically, and Sunday is the traditional day for that

AEROBIC EXERCISE

• *Running, biking or treadmill/stair-machine are the simplest forms of aerobic activity* - Running may have benefits over the others due to a more natural motion and because the slight jarring that occurs is said to help release toxins, settle the intestines and may help to keep joints well set - Running instead of using a machine also allows you to workout anywhere/anytime with only a pair of shoes

• Keeping with what some experts recommend, a *minimum of 20-25 minutes of aerobic activity* is needed to reach the fat-burning and heart-strengthening heart rate

After a few weeks of getting warmed up, **a distance of about 2-2.5 miles should be easily completed within the 20-25 minute time frame**

• Back stretches and abdominal exercises are on aerobic workout days following the more intense aerobic activity

We need to put the right foods inside of us in order to get the nutrition, or chemical energy, that our body needs for all of its functions. The kinds of food eaten should also have the physical properties that help to maintain a strong metabolism and digestive system. In addition to chemical energy (fats, carbohydrates, and protein) and needed nutritional compounds (like minerals, enzymes, and antioxidants), the body needs fiber to keep the intestines clear and needs foods that are digestible so that compounds will make it into the blood stream and eventually reach the organs and tissues that need it. Therefore, it is crucial to fill our diet with foods that are natural and have a concentrated amount of the things that our bodies need, and avoid those that are naturally foreign to our bodies and are chemically lacking in the things that feed our bodies.

Eating the proper foods also leads to having an attractive physique because your body will not be hindered from processing foods nor from cleaning itself of unwanted toxins which affect organ function and metabolic rate. Putting the right foods into your body will prevent the storing of disproportionate amounts of fat in the wrong places and will assure the growth of a healthy amount of muscle mass, which also creates an attractive proportion and keeps fat-burning going strong, thus keeping body fat percentage under control.

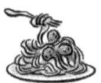 **MEAL SIZE AND FREQUENCY**

• It has been suggested that the body digests and metabolizes food better if it is eaten in 5-6 smaller meals per day rather than our current tradition of 3 meals per day - however, this is an ideal and is not very practical since frequent meals can become a distraction from living life

> It is much more convenient and still very much effective to simply **keep the modern tradition of eating 3 full meals per day**, being careful to maintain the use of good quality food, and the need for additional meals will be unnecessary

• A key to maintaining a fat-burning metabolism is to eat enough food during your meal to satisfy you (in terms of quantity *and* quality) and then to *not eat between meals* - this period of letting your digestive system lie fallow for a period helps to keep it in better health and embracing the feeling of hunger until the next meal helps to keep the metabolism high, thus allowing it to enter a fat-burning phase

• If hunger is a problem, it is easy to prepare for up to *2-3 snacks per day by carrying portable snacks with you* or having them close at hand at home as specifically-designated snack items

As stated above, modern food production does not always provide enough nutrition to get all we need in only 3 meals, due to poor food quality, so snacks or supplements can be helpful

FOOD TYPES AND PORTIONS

• Each meal should have a balance of **protein, vegetables, starch, fiber and fats, with fruit as a finisher** - all of these are needed in our diet and there is no way to get these things into our system except by paying close attention to what we are eating and *looking for each of these items* as we prepare for a given meal

• One expert suggests a fist-sized portion of each for a given meal, but this turns out to be too much food and is difficult to finish - nutritional needs are different between persons and even for the same person over periods of time, so portion size should vary as your bodily needs and appetite fluctuate

The exact portion size in a given meal is something more intuitive and must be developed over time by conscious awareness of yourself and what you are eating, but **a good rule-of-thumb for a portion size is about** *one cup, or 8 oz, for each type of food*

• When you are eating food that is healthy and natural, there is less concern over eating too much, particularly when it comes to consumption of fruits and vegetables, so concern over portion is not a major one in this diet plan

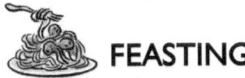

FEASTING

• It is good in life to truly enjoy oneself and to feel that a sea of good-ness surrounds you. *Feasting is a way to learn that sense of satisfac-tion and contentment that comes from truly immersing oneself in the goodness of life.* Plus, you have the opportunity to allow your body to experience a wider variety of foods, and in greater quantities, than during the week when the focus is more on discipline.

Being respectful of your body, what you eat and how much you eat is something that should not be neglected any day of the week - *Respecting the body's limits and needs is still im-portant even when feasting*, but the limits can be stretched in a way that is healthy and life-giving

• **Feast one day per week, Saturday night into Sunday night being the traditional day.** Eat sweets and fatty foods or other foods that you enjoy that you don't eat during the week

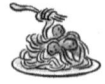

SAUCES
• **Sauces can add nutritional value, and lots of flavor** - mayonnaise, olive oil, apple cider vinegar, hommus, ketchup and mustard, spa-ghetti sauce, salad dressing and others can make a meal much more enjoyable and flavorful - have them as a regular part of meals

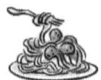

NATURAL FOODS ARE THE KEY
• It is the fresh, natural foods that contain all of the vitamins, antioxi-dants, and enzymes that your body needs in addition to the energy that the food supplies - EATING FOOD IS NOT ABOUT ENERGY ALONE - there is no way to get the nutrients that your body needs except by consuming them, one way or another

If you don't eat foods that get you the compounds that your body needs, then your only other option is to take supple-ments, or to remain less healthy

• Natural foods, sometimes called "whole" foods, are foods that are in the state that they would be found when in their natural environ-ment - examples of whole foods would be:

An apple that was not treated with herbicides and so has its *natural enzymes* still on the skin that help to properly digest the fruit and help to transport nutrients from the apple around the body

A ribeye steak that comes from a cow that has not been treated with hormones nor has been processed with flavorings or preservatives, and so has the *chemical properties* that it had when it was cut from the untreated cow

• It is not always possible to get whole foods because so few stores actually provide foods that are not altered in some way physically or chemically by how they are grown, processed and shipped

Usually the best you can do is get whatever slightly deficient foods the local grocery store provides, **eating as much fresh food instead of processed foods as possible, and then adding supplements to the diet**

If you are lucky, then you have a few options other than your local grocery store, such as a *farmer's market, a food co-op, or one of the few chains that provides non-processed foods*

• The things that fresh, natural foods provide that cannot be found in foods that provide mere energy are:

B-Vitamins: Riboflavin, niacin, thiamine
Anti-oxidants: Vitamins A, C, E
Fiber: Mostly in the form of cellulose from fruits & vegetables
Minerals: Iron, Zinc, Magnesium
Electrolytes: Sodium, Potassium
Enzymes: e.g., lactase, found in untreated milk, helps to digest the sugar naturally found in the milk

• One of the most important reasons to try to get as much of the vitamins you need from the food you eat, even instead of supplements, is that natural foods provide the chemical substances that your body needs in the *proper proportion*, in a form that is *soluble* in your system and that comes along with the *enzymes and other natural compounds* needed to digest the energy in the food and to absorb the vitamins and minerals

SUPPLEMENTS

• Supplements can be taken for specific vitamins & minerals, antioxidants, enzymes and the like - some experts say that food these days is lacking in nutrients, likely due to artificially growing mass quantities of larger than normal fruits, vegetables, meats and grains

Supplements are best taken daily, in proper proportion - Without doing excessive reading about daily nutritional needs, you can look for the items listed above, with a focus on finding products that are:

> Soluble - The vitamin/mineral is able to be absorbed by the body very well because it is *in a form that is natural to the body*

> Complete - Sometimes there are *multiple compounds needed together* to get full absorption and full effect and often times these are neglected for a more easy to manufacture product

> Specific - A single daily multi-vitamin tablet is not very effective because in order to get such a variety of chemically active substances into the same pill, they have to give you a modified version of each - So *get one B-Vitamin supplement, one Anti-Oxidant supplement, etc.* And they will be more chemically effective

> Proportional - You don't need several 100% or several 1000% of the daily amount of a given nutrient in a day - you can find a supplement that gives a good balance of a few things together for a daily intake

FOODS TO AVOID

• Some foods are hard to digest, some have little nutritional value and others have substances that are foreign to our bodies and to natural food, such as chemicals or additives. For these reasons, it is generally good to do the following:

1. **Avoid excessive amounts of wheat and processed sugar**; they have little nutritional value and do not digest properly, they may even leach nutrients out of your body due to their chemically deficient characteristics

2. **Stay away from foods with preservatives, dyes, sweeteners, or artificial flavorings;** these are usually designed for some purpose other than providing nutrition and thus can actually interfere with the absorption of needed compounds

3. **Do not eat fast foods whatsoever**, even a pre-made sandwich from the local grocery store is better for you than fast food, and it can tide you over until you can get home to eat - if you consider it to be an occasional treat, it will not kill you, but if it becomes a habit it can undo the progress in health you have made

4. Go for **fresh foods instead of processed or packaged goods**; packaged foods not only tend to have chemicals and additives, but are also usually processed in such a way that they lose their nutritional value and do not digest properly, making them nutritionally almost useless

5. Get a **de-chlorination filter** for your tap water - chlorine kills healthy bacteria in our digestive systems, which is why it is a good disinfectant, but it is also a harsh chemical foreign to the body

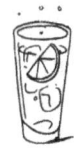

WATER CONSUMPTION
• One of the simplest and most crucial ways to keep general health and keep your metabolism at a high, fat-burning rate is to make sure you drink a sufficient amount of water everyday. It is the fuel that keeps your blood flowing and keeps your metabolism, which is a water-based system, running strong. Nutrients cannot get to your tissues and organs, toxins cannot be flushed, and body systems cannot operate properly without the needed amount of water in your body.

The FDA recommends drinking about 64 oz. per day, which is about 4 pints - However, after some experimentation it seems that only 4 pints a day, especially when exercising daily, is *not enough to keep the body hydrated*

Six pints per day creates a bloated feeling, like the body is flooded with water and somewhat depleted of energy due to the flushing out of nutrients in *excessive urination*

• **The best amount of water for your daily needs is 5 pints a day.** One pint of water should be consumed at each of the following times of day:

- **When you first wake up**, to get the blood flowing and to get the energy level high
- **Right after your morning workout,** to replenish fluid lost as sweat
- **Immediately after each of your three meals,** to help the nutrients get around your body

• It is handy to have a **one-pint glass** that can be used specifically for downing a quick pint when it is time. At first you will feel that you are forcing yourself to drink a little more water than your appetite wants, but after a while when you start to notice how much better you feel, you will see that *sometimes you have to be the master of your body and do what is best for it even when it seems to want otherwise.*

For the sake of simplicity and efficiency, the goals listed earlier in the booklet were sought in the selection of exercises:

1. Working **all** of the major muscle groups in a **balanced** way
2. Working as **many** muscles as possible in as **few** exercises as possible
3. **Not overworking** any muscle group by working it more than once in a pronounced way.
4. Needing only **one set of dumbbells** and no machines or special equipment
5. Using **normal movements** of the joints and muscles involved for ease of form and to avoid unhealthy strain on muscles and joints

==>Targeted Muscle Groups

Generally, it is easiest to target each muscle group by selecting one exercise for each muscle group. Some muscle groups will be worked secondarily by a given exercise and so do not need to be targeted directly, such as the tricep muscle. The biceps are worked in several exercises, but are also targeted by a specific exercise because biceps are generally desired to be strong.

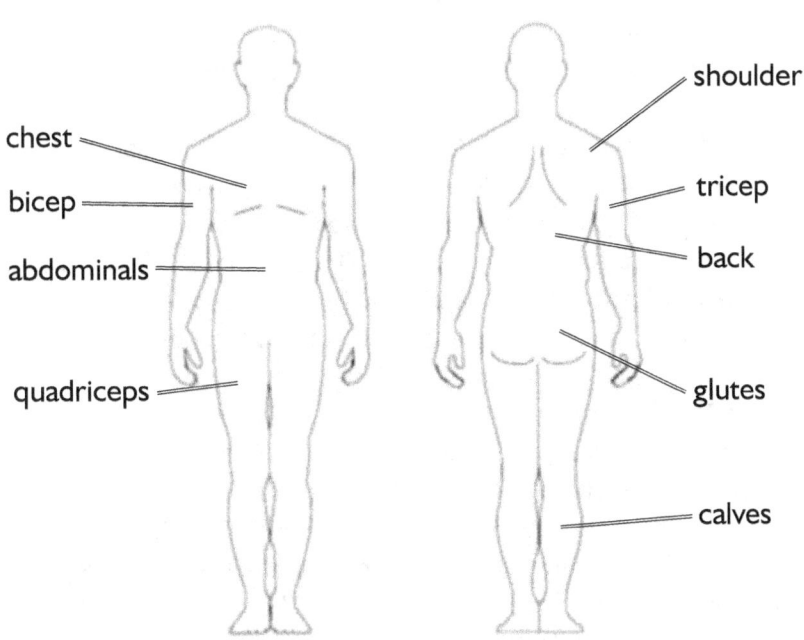

==>Specific Exercises of the Plan

The stretches were chosen so that the entire body could be stretched in only two stretches. The bend over stretch stretches the entire body to one degree or another. For the upper body routine, as few exercises as possible were chosen to target each of the major muscle groups. Back exercises were chosen to stretch and strengthen the back and torso in all directions. The lower body workout was designed to strengthen the major leg muscles and the lower abdomen and ankles. All exercises below are on pp.26-44 in the order shown here.

STRETCHING (Daily)
1. Bend Over & Reach - 3 times x 20 seconds (forward & backward)
2. Calf Stretch - 3 times x 20 seconds

UPPER BODY (Monday and Friday)
1. Push-Up (chest, triceps) - 3 sets x 20 repetitions
2. Bent Over Row (back, triceps) - 3 sets x 20 repetitions
3. Front Raise (shoulder) - 3 sets x 20 repetitions
4. Biceps Curl (biceps) - 3 sets x 20 repetitions
5. V-Raise (shoulder) - 3 sets x 20 repetitions
6. Seated Back Raise (lower back) - 3 sets x 20 repetitions

BACK/ABDOMEN (FOLLOWING AEROBIC - Tue, Thu, Sat)
1. Diagonal Stretch (back) - 3 sets x 20 seconds (each combination)
2. Hip Flexor (glutes) - 3 sets x 20 seconds
3. Torso Rotation (back)- 3 sets x 20 repetitions (10 times each side)
4. Neck & Back Stretch (upper back) - 3 times x 20 seconds
5. Regular Crunch (abdominals) - 3 sets x 20 repetitions

LOWER BODY (Wednesday)
1. Squat (quadriceps) - 3 sets x 20 repetitions
2. Calf Raise (calves) - 3 sets x 20 repetitions
3. Side Lift (lateral leg muscles) - 3 sets x 20 repetitions
4. Tilted Back Crunch (lower abdominals) - 3 sets x 20 repetitions
5. Knee-to-Chest (upper abdominals) - 3 sets x 20 repetitions
6. Ankle Alphabet (ankle tendons) - 3 sets x 20 repetitions
7. Seated Back Raise (lower back) - 3 sets x 20 repetitions

==>Movement Basics

There is a basic way of moving the joints and limbs during weight-lifting exercises that helps to protect the joints and puts the emphasis of the weight on the muscles instead. Injury to joints is probably the main negative effect of weight-lifting for which to keep an open eye. The following few points can help to ensure safe and enjoyable time spent with the dumbbells to be used in the exercises:

1. Keep Joints close to a 90-degree angle - Probably the most helpful way to protect joints when lifting weights is to try to keep the elbows at nearest a 90-degree angle during the entire movement of the weight. This usually means sticking the elbows out a bit to the sides while performing the exercise. This angle between your limbs allows your muscle to be the one responsible for holding the weight of your dumbbell, instead of a straighter angle, which puts the emphasis on the joints. Intentionally stick the elbows out a bit in a natural way as you perform each of the upper body exercises.

2. Focus on using the target muscle - Focus on squeezing the muscle that you are targeting by the exercise you are doing. This requires some effort of mind, but mostly it requires that you simply put your focus on what you are doing. The focus of any physical movement is on how you are moving your body. Focus on the speed and form as you put your mind on the muscle you are squeezing.

So if, for example, you are doing a bicep curl, which is an arm exercise, you should not be using a back muscle excessively during the repetition. Likewise, if you are doing a push-up, which is a chest exercise, you should not be flexing your abdominal muscles too much - they should be firm and stable while you push yourself upward using your chest muscles.

3. Pause for one second at each end of the repetition - This is a way to make sure that you are not moving the weight too erratically or too quickly so that you get the slow, careful motion that gives good muscle-building resistance. Move thoughtfully; not particular-ly slow, but slower than if you were rushing through the routine.

4. Be aware of any excessive joint pain - It is likely that your joints will feel like they have been used more than is comfortable, and they may feel a little fiery pain, but it should be nothing sharp or rough or grinding. The weights should be light enough to avoid this. If sharp pain persists, see your physician or consider discon-tinuing the workout routine. SORENESS OF MUSCLES IS EX-PECTED, RESIDUAL PAIN AT A JOINT, OR COMPLETE INABILITY TO MOVE IS NOT OK.

==>Running Form

There are different ways of running, but there is a particular way of running that helps to protect the joints and puts the weight of your body on the mus-cles in your legs instead of on the joints in your legs. **The basic idea is to keep the elbows and knees bent with a 90-degree angle in mind as if you are**

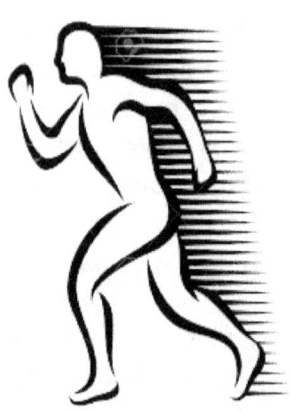

sitting in an arm chair. This allows your leg mus-cles to be flexed and hold the tension caused by moving your legs forward. And keeping your el-bows bent helps to create good momentum when you swing them forward to counterbalance your leg movements. You should push off of your toes a little bit with each stride in order to activate your calf muscle. The leg position will feel a little bit awkward because you will not be taking long strides, but instead will take smaller steps that will also have a little more bounce.

==>Breathing

1. When doing exercises - **Keep a rhythm to your breathing.** Breathe **out** during exertion and breathe **in** when returning weight to resting position. Take about 10 deep breaths between sets. This gives oxygen to the muscles.
2. When running - **Also keep a rhythm to your breathing.** It does not need to be overly controlled, but it should be *intentional.* Some control, some flow.

The most important factor in the success of the diet plan is the consumption of natural foods. This means primarily keeping the major categories of foods in each meal. Buying fresh meats, fruits, and vegetables and good quality breads and nuts are essential to the nutritional aspects of the diet plan. The next most important part of the plan is to make sure to eat the proper proportion of each category in each meal. The options are meant to be obvious.

Meat - Organic meats are best, but are somewhat expensive so ordinary good quality meats may be more cost-effective

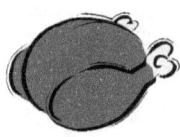

-You can find good quality meat distributors who sell meats that are visibly more natural and have the red color and the texture that accompanies meat from naturally-fed and naturally-tended animals

-Meat from high-production farms have a pinker meat instead of a red meat and have a pasty pale fat instead of a firmer white fat
-Beef, chicken, pork or other typical meats are ok

Starch - The best starches are probably yams or other tubers, a good quality rice, or a whole grain bread
-Look for the best product you can find, that which looks most natural and has the imperfections that reveal that it has not been overprocessed -A whole grain bread that is good quality will have a heartyness and weight to it, not like a bread that has finely-processed flour

Vegetables/Fruit - Look for ones that have imperfections and strong odors and colors, these are the things that reveal naturally grown produce - they are less perfect looking, more organic or freely grown - they have variation in color and texture
-Canned, fresh, or frozen fruit is good
-Salads are a particularly good idea because you get a variety of different vegetables - try to be creative and generous...lots of vegetables is better than few...have multiple types of lettuce, avoid iceberg, which is only filler and have at least about 5 or more vegetables

Nuts - Cashews, Almonds, and raw mixed nuts are the best kinds for both fiber and healthy proteins and fats, peanuts are just a filler

THE SAMPLE WEEKLY SCHEDULE IS KEY!

Having a sample schedule for the week can help to keep the Diet Plan and Workout Plan effectively. A sample schedule is as follows:

	Mon	Tue	Wed	Th	Fri	Sat	Sun
6 am	Morning Stretch (*then workout*)...						
	Upper	Aerobic	Lower	Aerobic	Upper	Aerobic	Rest
7 am	Breakfast...						
8 am	Work..						
6 pm	Dinner..						
10 pm	Bed...						

A sample menu for a day would be:

Breakfast - I portion meat - 3 eggs, with mayonnaise
　　　　　　 I portion starch - english muffin (if desired), with real butter
　　　　　　 3 veggies - celery, carrots, tomatoes - with ranch dressing
　　　　　　 I piece of fruit - banana
　　　　　　 I handful nuts - fancy mixed nuts

Lunch - I portion meat (left over from dinner), or sandwich (meat & cheese)
　　　　　 I portion starch - Handful whole grain crackers, chips and hummous
　　　　　 3 veggies - carrots, broccoli, parsnip
　　　　　 I piece of fruit - apple w/ peanut butter
　　　　　 I handful of nuts

Dinner - I portion meat - steak w/ worchestershire sauce on it
　　　　　 I portion starch - I cup of rice, w/ butter
　　　　　 3 veggies - yam, peas, tomatoes
　　　　　 I piece of fruit - peach
　　　　　 I handful nuts

Each portion being about 8 oz. or one cup
Meat can be portioned by weight, typically an 8 oz steak is best

Foods List & Other Notes

Meat - Beef steaks, pork steaks/chops/tenderloin, ground beef/meat, ham, chicken, beef/pork ribs, salmon, venison, lamb, tilapia

Starch - Whole grain wheat bread, spelt bread, sprouted grain breads

Fruits/Vegetables - Apples, bananas, pears, peaches, oranges, starfruit, mango, melons, tomatoes, carrots, beets, celery, mustard greens, eggplant…select as wide a variety as you can of what looks *potent*

Nuts - Almonds, cashews, fancy mixed nuts, pistachios

The foods that you select for your meals <u>do not</u> need to be limited to the above list. This is not a specifically tailored diet for one specific goal. You can eat what you want. <u>Natural is the key.</u>

•You will have to **use a little judgment** based on what makes you feel full, but generally round up - 6-8 oz of meat is good, but you can't overdo fruit and vegetables very easily…fruit varies by size and type

•You will want to have a **bowel movement** after each meal…3 times per day
-It not only can be done, but it becomes the norm after a while - go with the flow…Your stool should be brown and solid after a few weeks, which reveals your overall health level.

•The **basic dietary needs are protein, carbohydrates, and fat**
-Each handful is meant to provide one of each of these
-Fats are best added as fat on meat, or in sauces like mayonnaise
-Carbs are best found in starches or nuts and occasional snacks

•**Snacks** can be a great way to supplement meals throughout the day. The best way to provide snacks for yourself is to have some dried fruit and nuts on hand either at home, or with you at work so that you can grab a quick handful anytime. One snack = two handfuls.

•**You can add chips/cookies & other snacks**, but only after settled into the plan for a while to see what quantity & when to eat it
-Cookies and chips might be best only after dinner or only on week-ends, you can decide what to add after you get used to your own metabolism

The Crux of the Diet Plan

The crux of the **diet plan** is: <u>EMBRACING THE BURN</u> – which is LEARNING TO LIVE IN A CONSTANT STATE OF DESIRE

What you do is keep a more or less scheduled disciplined diet, and as a result you become accustomed to always having some unmet desire…

Simply not fighting against the returning hunger…entering into the abiding desire while keeping the commitment to snack only once between meals

The way that it bears fruit in your life is you learn to be free from feeling like you have to fulfill that desire immediately or fully

Self-control, temperance, strength of will and emotional freedom all come from the diet plan

The Crux of the Workout Plan

The crux of the **workout plan** is <u>KEEPING MOVING</u> - ACTUALLY WILLING THE LIFE THAT YOU HAVE FOR YOURSELF…starting with discipline

Not only must you keep moving through the difficulty of weight resistance, of establishing a new routine and of trying to see how this plan fits in your life, but you also reach the point where you feel you've got the motivation to get things done, to accomplish things in life

And now there is a clean slate for the day to work with and the same initiative that was used doing the workout can be harnessed to do whatever other business needs to fit into your schedule

You will also have the psychological and emotional strength to focus on the tasks that you have to perform each day, and you will have the confidence to believe that you can carry out, and follow through with, your responsibilities and desires

Sleep - Some have said that 1.5 hr sleep cycles is best…9 hrs seems to be too much and 6 hrs seems minimal, so *7.5 hrs may be ideal*
- A 0.5 hr nap in the afternoon is said to be as much as 1.5 hrs at night, so you could sleep 6 hrs, take a 0.5 hr nap, and feel like you slept 7.5 hrs
- Sleep is crucial to maintaining good mental and physical health (a good supplement from *Whole Foods* is called "Restful Sleep")

Energy balance and energy economy - These are the focal points of this whole plan: Diet, Exercise, Sleep, Water…All are factors that affect the rate of metabolism & the functioning within a stable metabolic state. So what? *The human body and the human life are an economy of inputs & outputs -* The right balance produces fruitfulness and health

Recommended reading:

1. *Body for Life* - Bill Phillips…Designed a workout routine and principles for building a muscular physique. Very effective if your focus is on growing muscle mass more than general physical health
2. *Better Health Through Natural Healing* - Ross Trattler, N.D., D.O….Has a natural remedy for healing of many common conditions and diseases. A great resource for avoiding expensive medical tests or prescriptions every time that you have a minor health problem. Good for preventive health care.

Finding a store that sells good quality food can be difficult, but there are a few chains that exist now around the country that do. Some of these are *Trader Joe's* and *Whole Foods*. These chains are all around the country and they sell organic foods and foods that are free of preservatives, artificial flavors and colors or other additives. Good quality supplements from Trader Joe's that can get you started is:

       Joint Support - With MSM, Glucosamine, & Chondroitin
       Men's Formula - Contains multiple daily vitamins & minerals
       Calcium, Magnesium & Zinc
       Synergistic C - Vitamin C Complex
       High Potency B "50" - A supplement containing multiple B vitamins
       Super Green Drink - Powder, berry flavor - Contains many antioxidants and vitamins from dried and powdered fruits and vegetables

---

Warming up and cooling down before/after workouts - Normally, it is rec-
ommended that a warm up and cool down be done before and after each
workout. The morning stretch already accomplishes some of this, especially
if it is done slowly and intentionally. Typically, a 5-minute warm up is recom-
mended before workouts, but this can be time consuming and may not be
necessary. For the aerobic workout, simply walking for a few hundred yards
prior to starting jogging may be all that is needed to loosen up your muscles.
The jogging itself will stretch your muscles and loosen you up. *Unless you
are planning to run very fast as if training for a race, then you can do without
a serious warmup.* Likewise, with the upper body workout. *Simply performing the exercises slowly and intentionally will be enough to prevent injury and
will help stretch the muscles and increase blood flow.*

Vegetable and fruit washing - Since there are often chemicals and polishing
compound applied to the surface of produce sold in most stores today, it can
be desirable to purchase a fruit & vegetable washing solution that removes
the compounds applied to the surface of the produce. These chemicals are
sometimes petroleum-based or are adherents from the insecticide or herbi-
cide class of chemicals. A store like Trader Joe's has such produce washing
compounds, which are often citrus-based.

Alternative health aids (sauna, chiropractic care, etc.) - There are many
ways of maintaining good health that are only common in limited circles and
not in mainstream society, but which are very effective. Sitting in a sauna at
your local gym for a half-hour once per week can release many toxins and
relax your muscles making you feel light and fresh for the entire week. Chiropractic care is one of the primary sources of preventive health care, and
often whole food supplements that have healing properties are available
through practitioners offices as well. The functioning of organs, muscles and
other body systems depend on maintaining proper joint alignment so that
nerves are not pinched and can send signals effectively. Look up Dr. Potter
at Canton Center Chiropractic Clinic: www.cantoncenterchiropractic.com.

Meditation - One of the greatest benefits of the daily workout is that it can
be a time to clear the mind and to ponder things that are important, to tackle
practical concerns or discern life principles for how you want to live.

So the big question now is… "What do I do?"

FOLLOW THE WEEKLY SCHEDULE (p. 20)

…WHICH PRIMARILY MEANS DOING THE EXERCISES THAT PERTAIN TO EACH DAY (Upper on Monday, Aerobic on Tuesday…)

Also…
…GO GROCERY SHOPPING IN A DISCIPLINED WAY, PURCHASING SPECIFICALLY CHOSEN ITEMS THAT MATCH WITH THE PRINCIPLES
…COOK WHATEVER MEALS YOU WANT USING "NATURAL" FOODS
…ADD SNACKS IF SO DESIRED, PREFERABLY DRIED FRUIT & NUTS, UP TO THREE TIMES PER DAY

The best way to be effective each day is to:

1. **Stretch** - Following the two stretches on the following pages
2. **Do the day's workout** - Following the exercises listed on the following pages or the Running Form
3. **Mentally prepare your meals** for each day and gather what you need
4. **Carry snacks** with you or have them on hand at home

…AND ENJOY LIVING A HEALTHY LIFE!

S1 BEND OVER & REACH

3 sets x 20 seconds (forward, then backward)

This stretch involves bending over forward, touching the toes, holding for 20 seconds, and then bending over backward as far as possible, holding for 20 seconds. Bending over backward is awkward, but you can focus the tension of your stretch so that it works effectively on your muscles. *The goal is to stretch as many of the major body muscles as possible, which are on the front and back of the body, in one stretch.*

The best way to make this stretch effective is to *put the hands together, as if swimming*, and touch the floor, then direct that same V-shaped arm pattern behind your head, pointing behind you as far as you can reach as if you were pointing to an object behind you. Repeat the stretch three times for 20 seconds each direction.

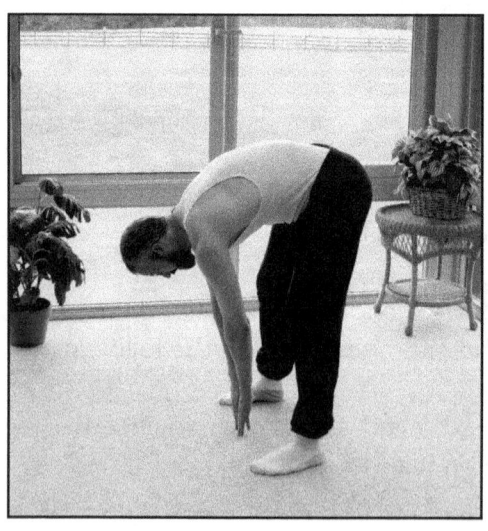

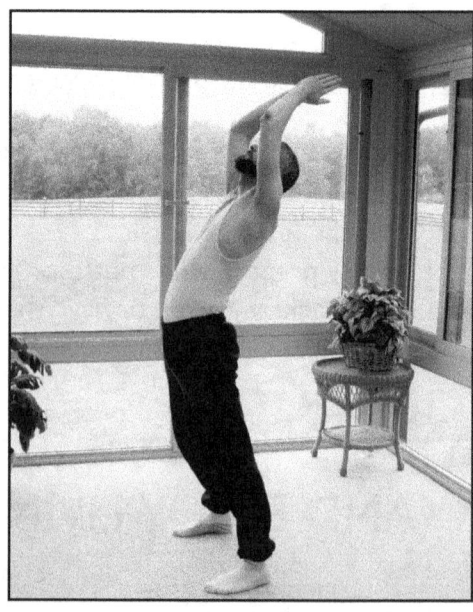

S2   CALF STRETCH

3 sets x 20 seconds

      This stretch involves standing on a step on the balls of the feet and allowing the heel to drop below the toes, holding for 20 seconds. This is most easily done on a staircase or a curb where there is an elevation difference that can be utilized. The goal is to feel tension in the muscle in the back of the lower leg especially just above the heel, since this muscle is one of the few not stretched by the bend over and reach stretch, which is a total body stretch.

      In the absence of a stair to stand on, the stretch can also be performed by leaning against a wall and flexing the ankle until the calf muscle is pulled tight. Simply lean against the wall forward, holding yourself up by your hands until the 20 seconds has passed, then repeat.

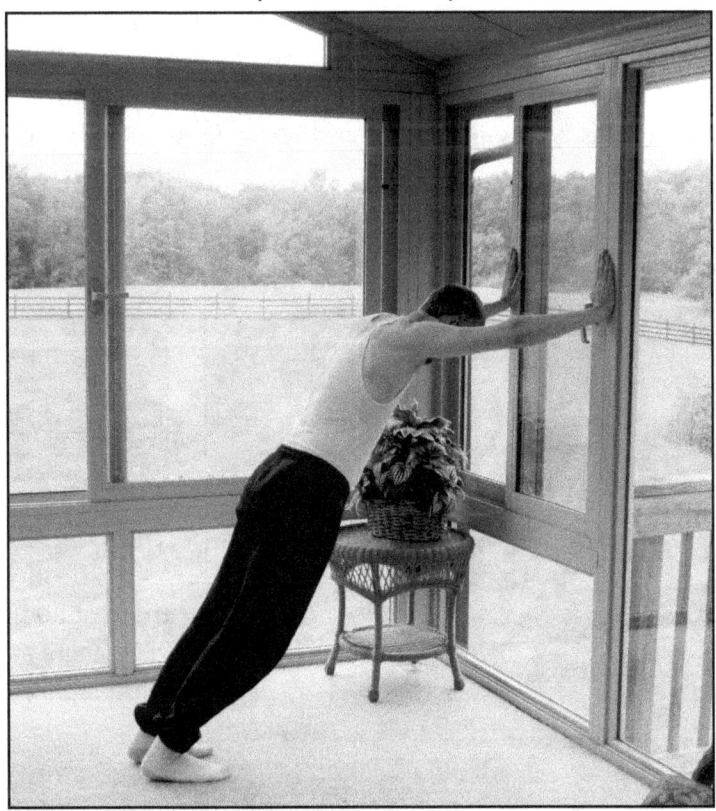

U1

PUSH-UP

3 sets x 20 repetitions

      The push-up is one of the simplest and most common exercises for the upper body. It is ideal because it uses only the body's own weight in order to create resistance. In order to get the maximum benefit from the exercise it is desirable to learn to perform it by lifting the entire body weight instead of only a partial body weight. If the exercise is too difficult at first, it can be performed by resting on bended knees, or if you are really weak at first, then you can do it by leaning against a wall. You should be able to reach the point where you can do your whole body after a few weeks of working out. The most important point for effectiveness is to keep the elbows pointed out away from the body, at roughly a 90-degree angle.

      It is likely in the first few weeks that the push-ups will be too difficult to finish all 20 repetitions of each set in one continuous set. You may have to stop and rest before finishing all 20 reps. You can break the 60 reps down into more sets, however, in order to work the upper body muscles enough to build muscle mass, you will have to resolve to finish all 60 repetitions in every workout.

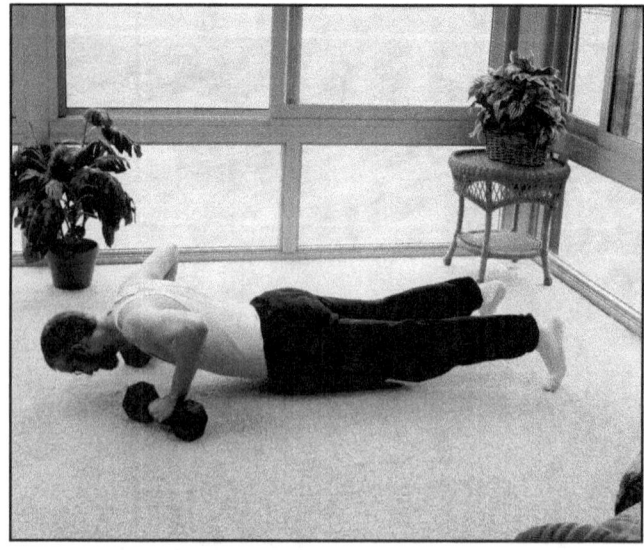

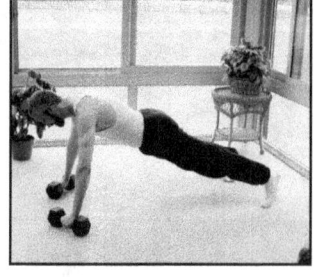

TIP: Use your weights to push off of – set them at about a 45-degree angle at shoulder width apart

U2   BENT OVER ROW

3 sets x 20 repetitions

The bent over row is aimed at exercising the back muscles, primarily. The hinge of the exercise is the prostrated posture that allows the back muscles to engage in a pulling motion toward the upper body as your arms lift the weight. The elbow points back behind the body and the line of movement of the weight is approximately along that line. The knees should be slightly bent and the back should be leaning over forward. The arms should pull the weight upward along the line of the thigh, which should be at close to a 45-degree angle from the floor.

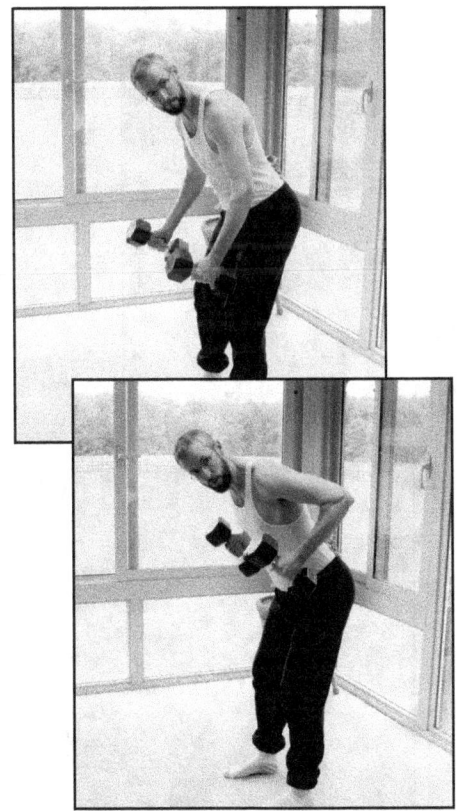
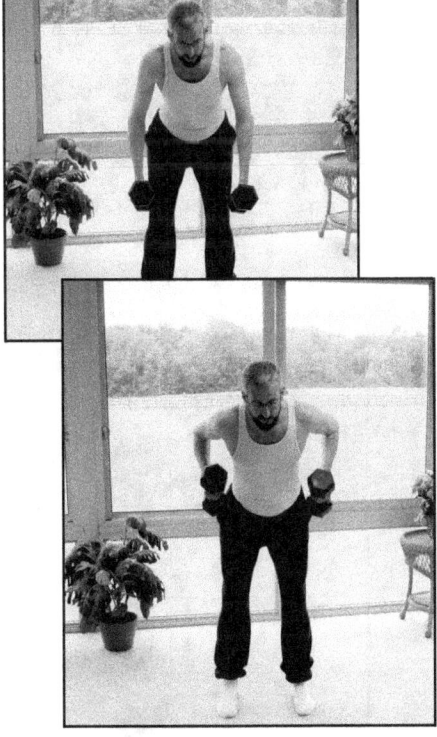

U3   FRONT RAISE

3 sets x 20 repetitions

The push-up and bent over row work the shoulder to a certain degree, however, the back of the shoulder does not get strengthened by either of those exercises. The front raise is a slightly unusual motion, but it accomplishes the necessary angle required to work the back of the shoulder. The most important part of the exercise is to keep the weight in front of the torso as you are lifting it. The mind should focus on squeezing the upper/back part of the shoulder and the back of the upper arm as the weight is lifted. The hands should be lifting up toward the shoulder from the resting position.

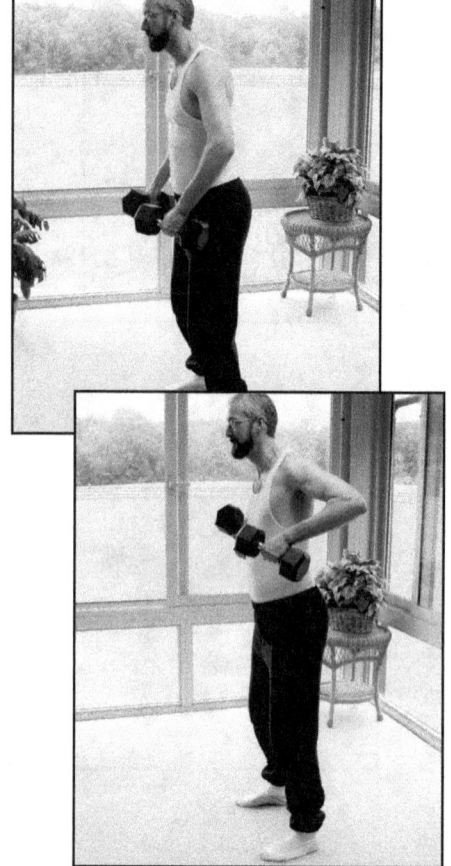
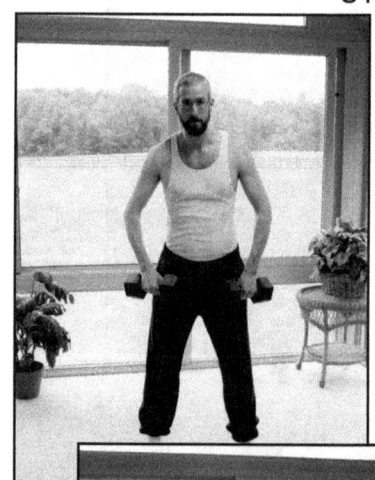
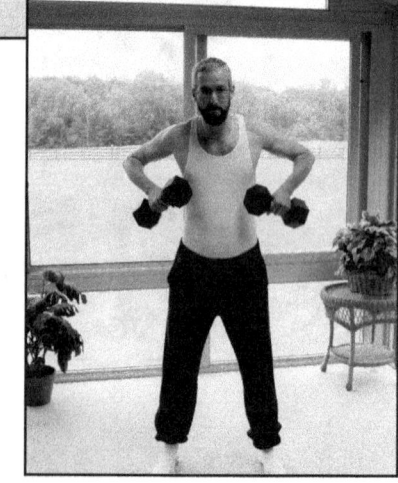

U4   BICEPS CURL

3 sets x 20 repetitions

Bicep curls are the most straight-forward way to strengthen the upper arm muscles. The goal is simply to lift the weight straight upward by bringing the lower arm up to meet the upper arm. The important part of making the exercise work is keeping the elbows stationary, just in front of your body, and keeping your back straight. The tendency with this exercise is to lean backward or to try to use your back muscles to finish the arm movement of the repetition. Doing either of these takes away from growing the arm muscles. Make sure the arm muscles are actually doing the work. One way to ensure this is to keep the range of motion small. Keep the weight always suspended by the arms, never letting the arms go completely limp and then stop the upward motion of the weight just before it reaches the vertical position and hold it there for a moment before letting it down again.

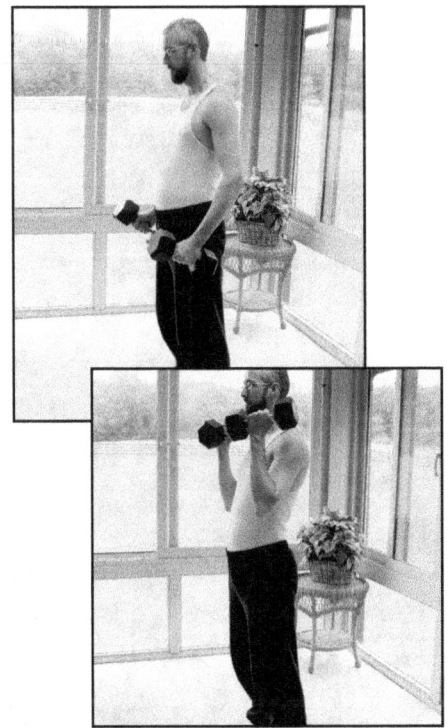

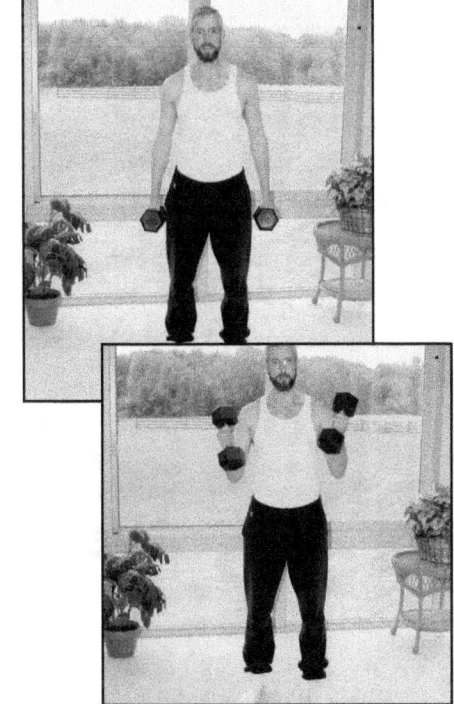

U5 V-RAISE

3 sets x 20 repetitions

Again, it is difficult to train the upper/back part of the shoulder, so the v-raises was adapted from a military workout to attack that part of the shoulder that is not easily strengthened. A particular benefit to this exercise is that it does not overly strain the rarely used shoulder muscles, but instead involves a motion that does not require a weight. This exercise should feel a little bit awkward because we are intentionally trying to move in a way we often do not.

The exercise is performed by holding the hands out slightly forward and to one side with the thumbs pointing upward. The motion is then to simply bring the hand and thumb upward while slightly rotating the arm up and over toward the back as you raise the hand. Basically, the hand is being lifted straight up into the air, as in a straight line vertically, while the angle of the arm slightly turns and twists to follow that line.

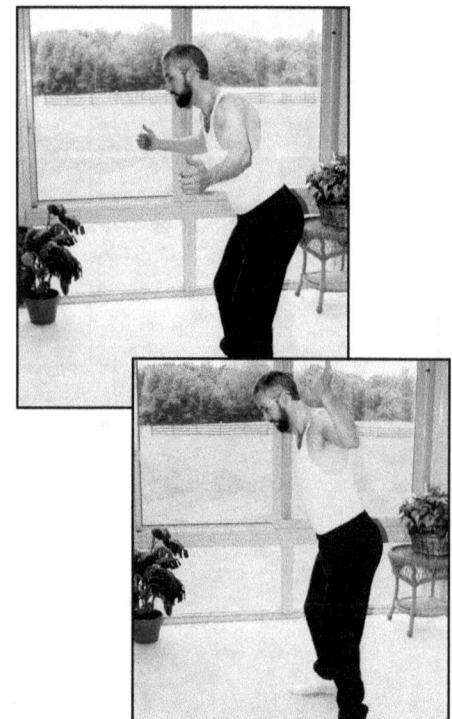
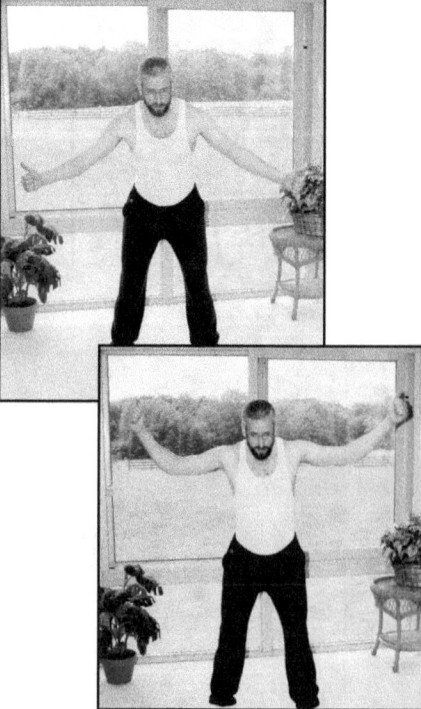

U6(L7)   SEATED BACK RAISE

3 sets x 20 repetitions

One of the easiest ways to strengthen the lower back is to sit in a chair and bend over, then sit upright. Do this repeatedly and it will make the lower back muscles stronger. This exercise does not require a weight and does not have a complicated form. Simply sit on the edge of a chair and repeatedly bend over and sit up again until all of the repetitions are completed. Rather than sitting on the ground in an awkward position, this approach emphasizes simplicity and ease of form. The back and head should be straight and the chest should bend in a nice circular arc down toward the knees, and then lift it up in exactly the same way, using the lower back muscles. It will be difficult until a few weeks have passed.

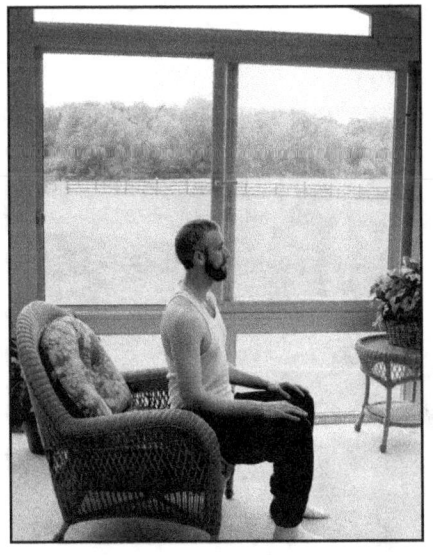

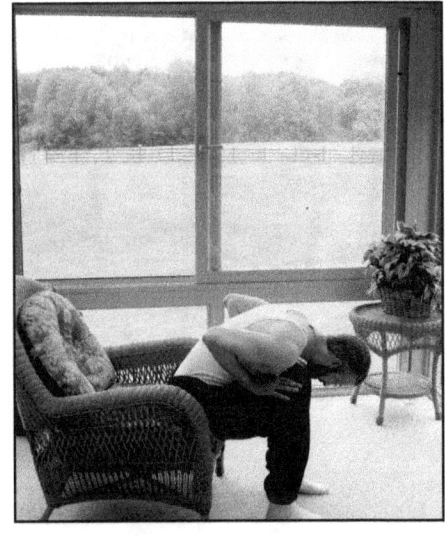

A 1   DIAGONAL STRETCH

3 sets x 20 seconds (each leg/arm combination)

The back is one area of the body that does often not get stretched except when performing some form of physical labor, but at that point it is often injured in some way also. Keeping the back stretched not only prevents joint and muscle injury but also allows greater flexibility and comfort when performing other activities, including sitting for long periods of time.

The way that this exercise is most effective is by extending the opposing arm and leg as far as possible in opposite directions, as if reaching for an object with your arm and pushing off of something with your leg. Do this with both sets of opposing arms and legs to keep the muscles in the middle of your back free from tension.

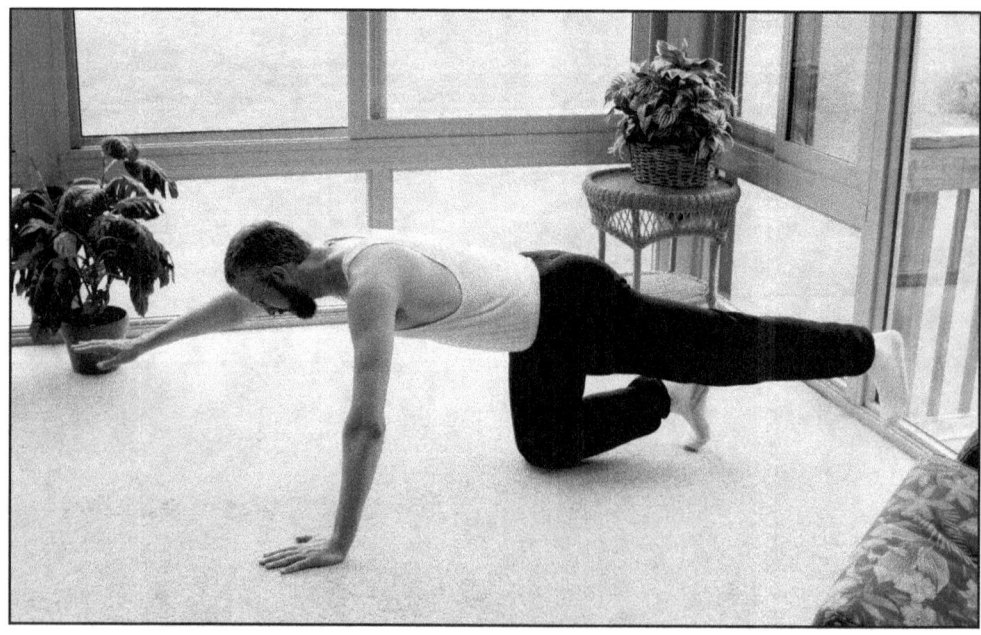

A2   HIP FLEXOR

3 sets x 20 seconds

The hip joints, like the back, are often not stretched until some physical labor is performed, at which time it is often already too late to prevent injury. They are a central joint that holds up the rest of the body weight and so they must be kept properly in place and functioning well. Running or doing other aerobic activity already stretches the hip joints and back, but an intentional strengthening of the muscles is well worth the little bit of extra effort in order to truly maintain proper functioning. The muscles in the buttocks are the primary ones that hold the hip joint in place and so they are targeted by flexing them and slightly pushing the hips in a backward motion behind the knees to create a point of tension, thus tightening the glutes in the rear. Do this and hold for 20 seconds, then repeat 3 times.

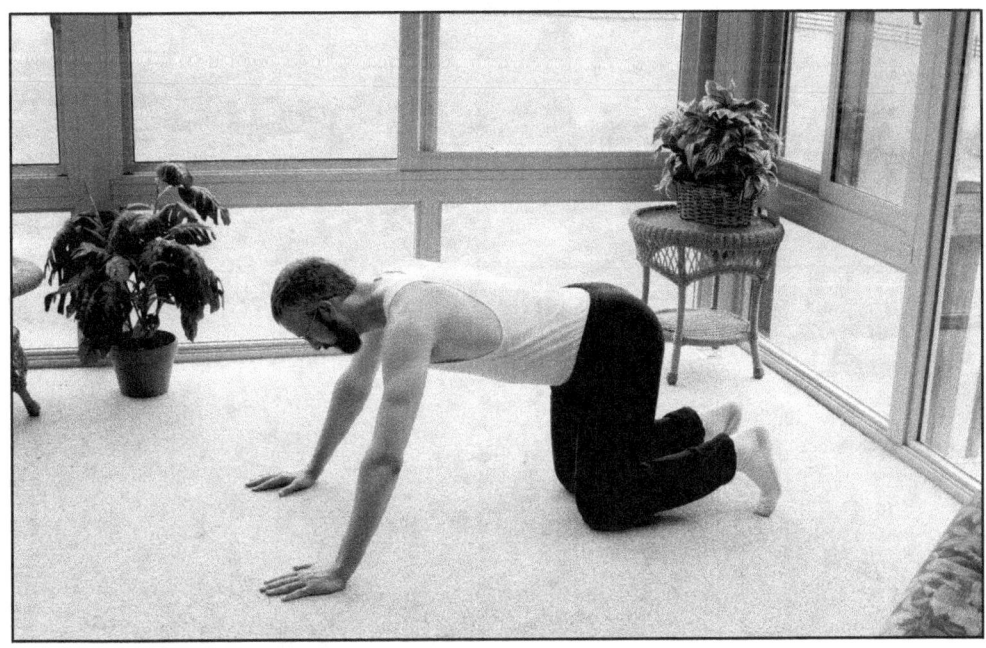

A3   TORSO ROTATION

3 sets x 20 repetitions (10 to left, 10 to right)

Stretching the torso can be done in a chair, but the emphasis some-times becomes shifted to the arms in an attempt to create the twisting force necessary to turn the torso effectively. It is much easier to lie on the floor and let the weight of the legs create the force needed to twist the torso from side to side. With arms folded on the stomach, the body can be turned com-pletely from one side to another from the waist down, while keeping the up-per body flat on the floor. The legs are best utilized by bending them at the knee and suspending them in the air as your turn them to either side.

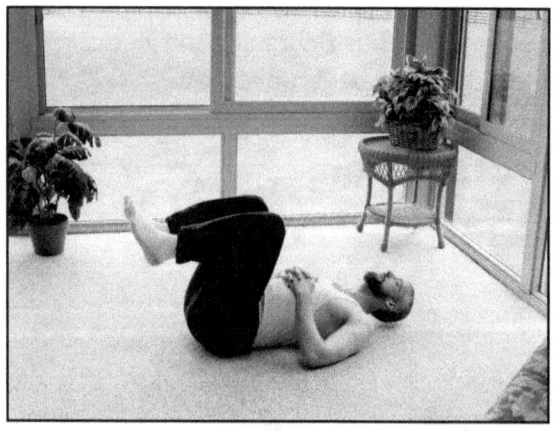

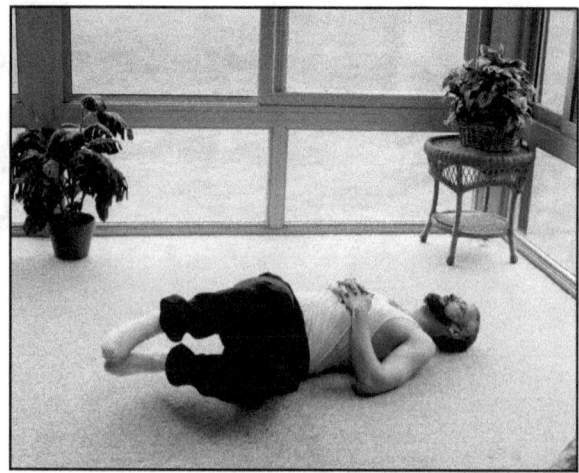

A4   NECK & BACK STRETCH

3 sets x 20 seconds

In order to stretch the muscles that are parallel to the spine, it is helpful to stretch the muscles in the back of the neck as well, to which they are also connected. As the torso stretch helps the middle back and the diagonal stretch helps the middle and lower back, this stretch helps the upper back and the muscles along the spine. The goal is to create tension along the axis of the spine by lifting the legs, reaching above the head with the arms and bending the head and neck forward.

Whereas the other back stretches focus on areas where there is movement, this exercise focuses on stretching the back itself as a structural unit. The hamstrings also receive some tension from raising the legs vertically, but the emphasis is felt most strongly at the neck and along the spine. Try to bring the head and legs as close together as possible when stretching.

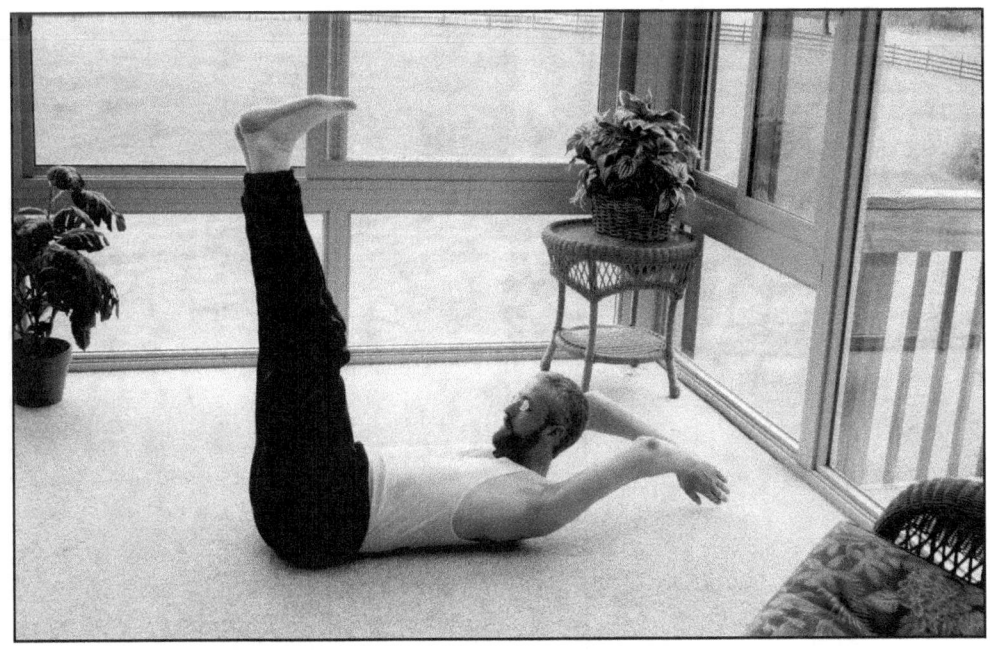

A5   REGULAR CRUNCH

3 sets x 20 repetitions

Regular crunches are the simplest way to strengthen the torso, front and back. Unlike sit-ups, the emphasis is not on moving the entire upper body off of the ground. Rather, it is only the shoulders that need to be lifted off the ground and toward the knees. The rest of the upper body remains in contact with the ground as the repetition is performed. The hands are held behind the head as the shoulders and upper torso are bent toward the knees, but only the upper abdominal muscles are squeezed during the movement.

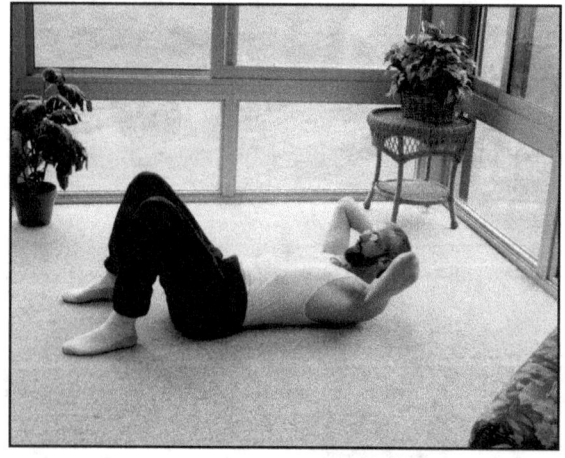

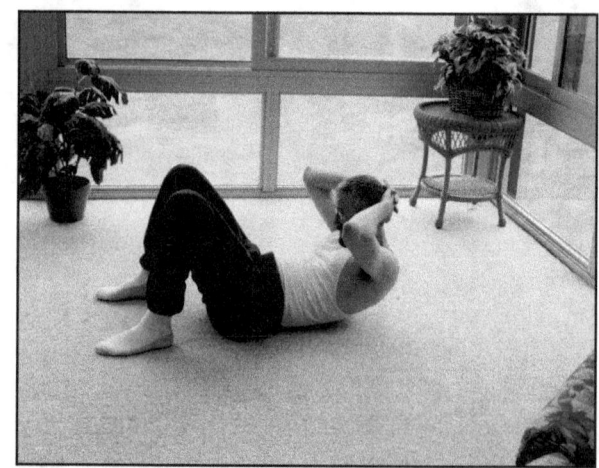

L I SQUAT

3 sets x 20 repetitions

The major muscle in the legs is the quadricep, or thigh muscle. This is the large muscle at the front of the leg used for kicking and for pushing up off the ground with the leg. A simple up and down motion is enough to stretch these muscles. Because the leg muscles are already big, we will avoid using additional weight and will simply focus on moving the body up and down with these muscles. Standing with feet shoulder width apart and with feet pointed slightly outward, turned about 30-degrees from forward, we can lower our entire body until our knees are bent to about 90-degrees and then raise it up again repeatedly. We emphasize our thigh muscle even more by keeping our back slightly curved with buttocks intentionally projecting rearward slightly.

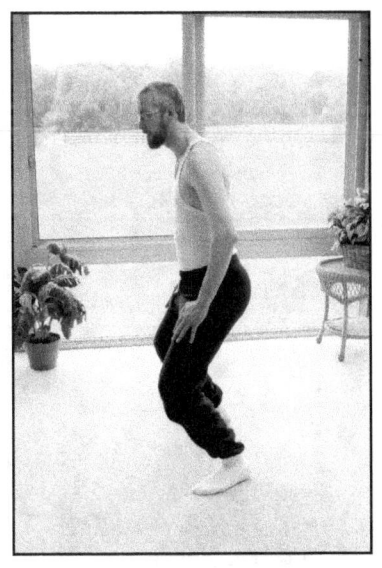
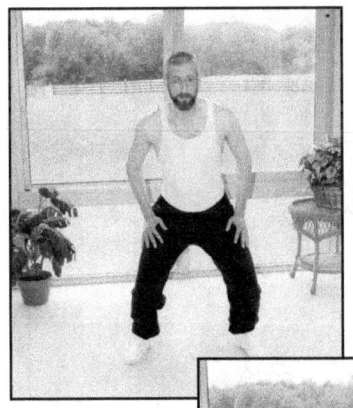

L2   SIDE LIFT

3 sets x 20 repetitions (each leg)

The outside of the leg is rarely worked by most activities unless there is frequent side-to-side movement, but because it is crucial to keeping the hip joint in place and moving smoothly, it is addressed in a specific exercise here. Standing stationary with one leg slightly more centered under the body, one leg is lifted and repeatedly directed up and to the side of the body. This is done with the knee slightly bent to help counteract the tendency to turn the leg outward and use the thigh muscle more than the hip muscle. Keeping the leg within the plane of the body, it can be moved at the hip in a circular motion, upward and then back down again.

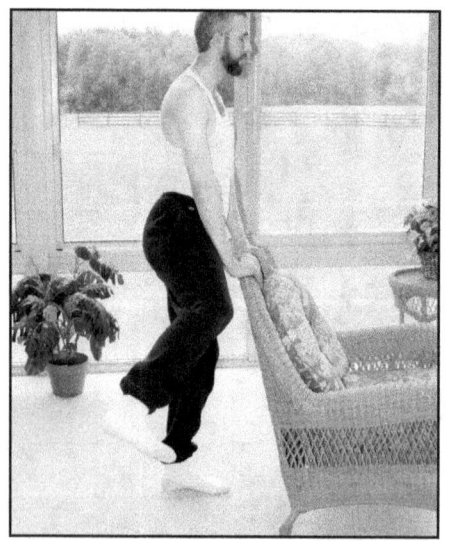

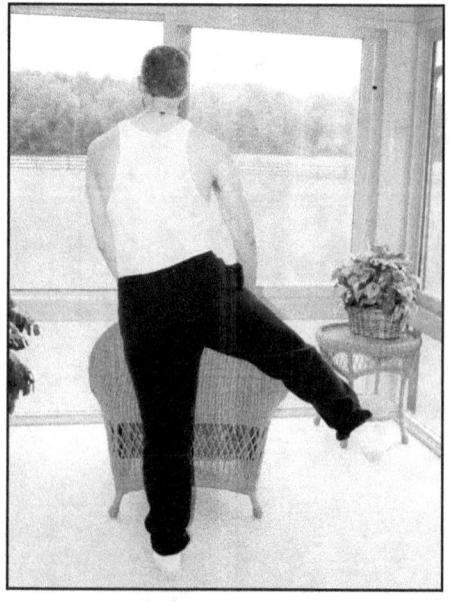

L3   CALF RAISE

3 sets x 20 repetitions (both legs together)

This exercise is very similar to the calf stretch. The same motion is used on an elevated step where the heel is dropped below the balls of the feet which are resting on the step. However, unlike the stretch, the emphasis here is on the exertion of lifting the entire body from the balls of the feet as they rest on the step. Each time the heel is lifted from below the balls of the feet to above, this is one repetition. The muscle in the rear of the lower leg which attaches to the heel is strengthened and becomes more tense. This allows greater force when jumping or when simply pushing off of one's feet when walking. The feet and calves are used all day when walking or standing and so are well worth keeping strong and toned.

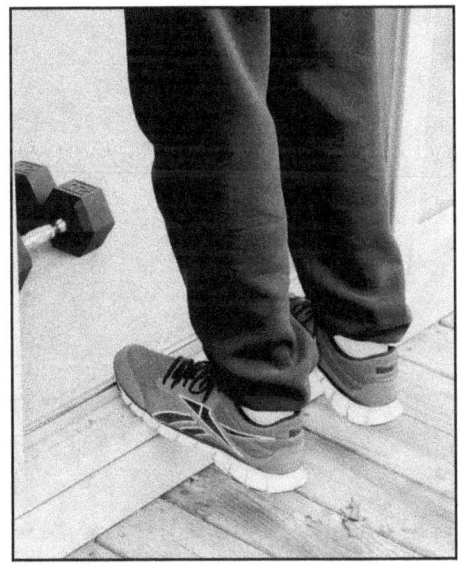

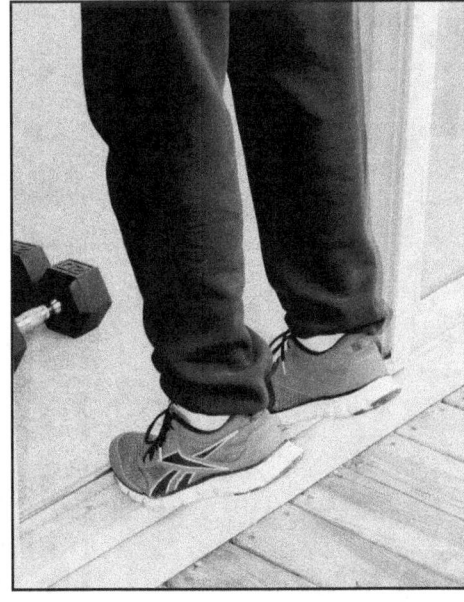

L4   TILTED BACK CRUNCH

3 sets x 20 repetitions

Tilted crunches are basically regular crunches except that the lower back is kept flat against the floor instead of allowing it to arch as it normally does when lying down. This flat position activates the lower abdominal muscles which are not worked as much during regular crunches. These crunches create additional strength for the torso and help to keep posture in a more erect position while walking, standing and sitting.

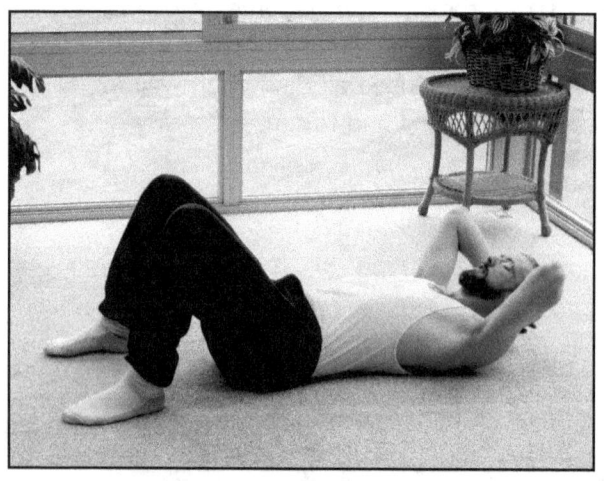

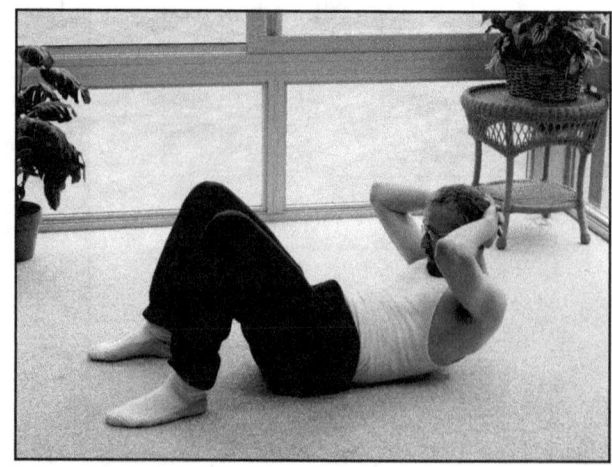

L5   KNEE-TO-CHEST

3 sets x 20 repetitions (both legs together)

This exercise adds strength to the torso by flexing the upper abdominal muscles, particularly where they attach to the rib cage. The legs are held together, bent at the knee and raised from the resting position until the upper thigh is touching the abdomen. This lifts the buttocks slightly off the ground but keeps the remainder of the upper body in the horizontal position on the floor during the repetition. This exercise stretches the lower back as it strengthens the abdomen.

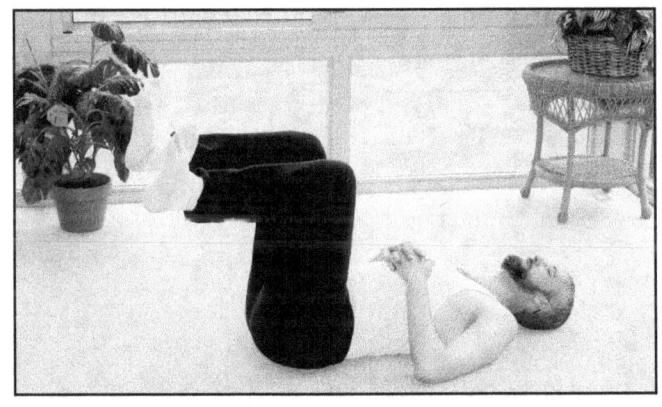

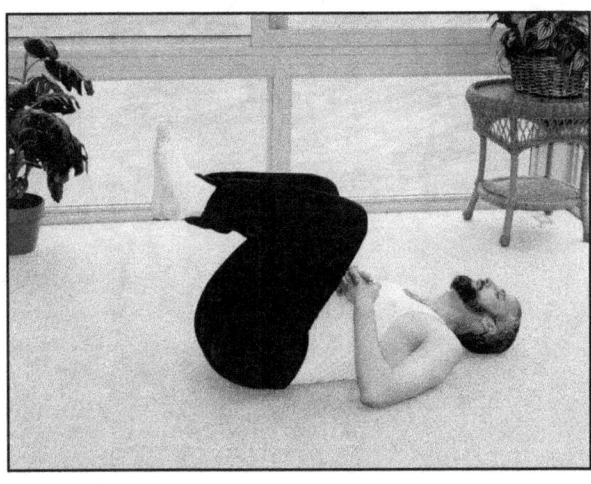

L6 ANKLE ALPHABET

3 sets (entire alphabet) x each leg

The thigh muscle and hamstring are worked during the squats; the calf muscle and side leg muscles are specifically targeted by other exercises, but the ankle muscles are left to be addressed. The best way to strengthen and stretch the ankle muscles is to move the ankle around in various directions. Tracing the alphabet with the toes is a way of moving the ankle in all directions and so is effective at keeping the ankle tendons stretched and toned. Point with the toes as if they were a pencil, drawing the lines of each letter. Trace the entire alphabet in the air, one time for each set, doing both legs simultaneously, moving the feet in opposite directions, e.g. Move both feet outward/inward at the same time, and up/down together.

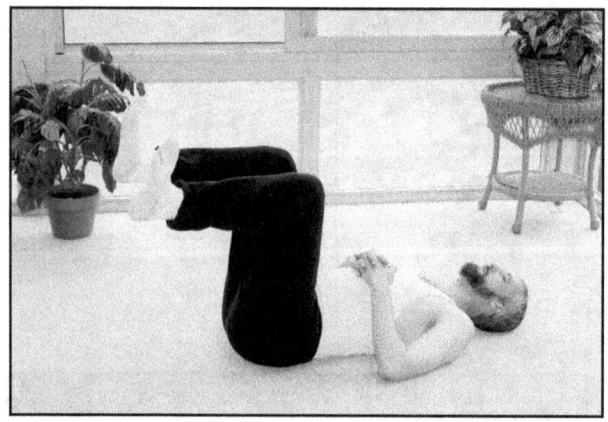

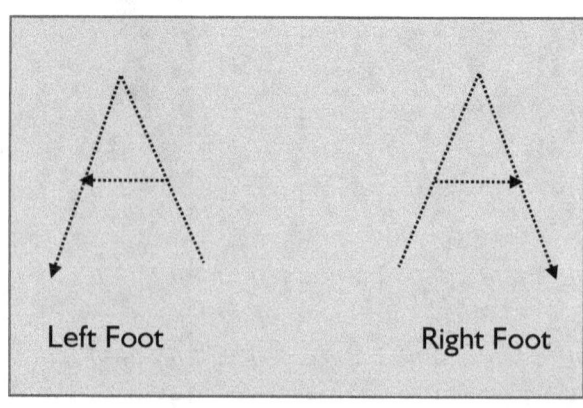

Left Foot   Right Foot